KURT RAY

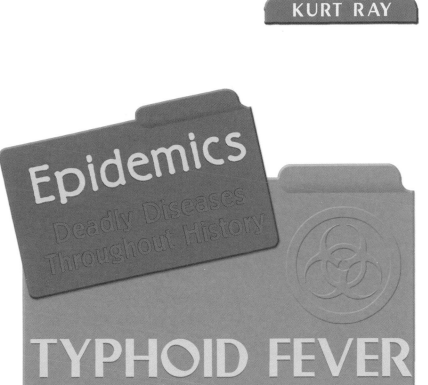

Epidemics
Deadly Diseases
Throughout History

TYPHOID FEVER

The Rosen Publishing Group, Inc.
New York

*For Matthew Curlewis*

Published in 2002 by The Rosen Publishing Group, Inc.
29 East 21st Street, New York, NY 10010

**Library of Congress Cataloging-in-Publication Data**

Ray, Kurt.
Typhoid fever / by Kurt Ray.
p. cm. — (Epidemics)
Includes bibliographical references and index.
ISBN 0-8239-3572-8 (lib. bdg.)
1. Typhoid fever—Juvenile literature. [1. Typhoid fever.
2. Diseases.]
I. Title. II. Series.
RA644.T8 R39 2001
614.5'112—dc21

2001002703

**Cover image:** An electron micrograph of the rod-shaped *Salmonella typhi* bacteria, which causes typhoid fever.

*Manufactured in the United States of America*

# CONTENTS

Introduction 5

Chapter 1 What Is Typhoid Fever? 8

Chapter 2 Centuries of Disease 18

Chapter 3 The Story of
Typhoid Mary 32

Chapter 4 In Search of a Cure 39

Chapter 5 A Future
Without Typhoid? 51

Glossary 57

For More Information 59

For Further Reading 61

Index 62

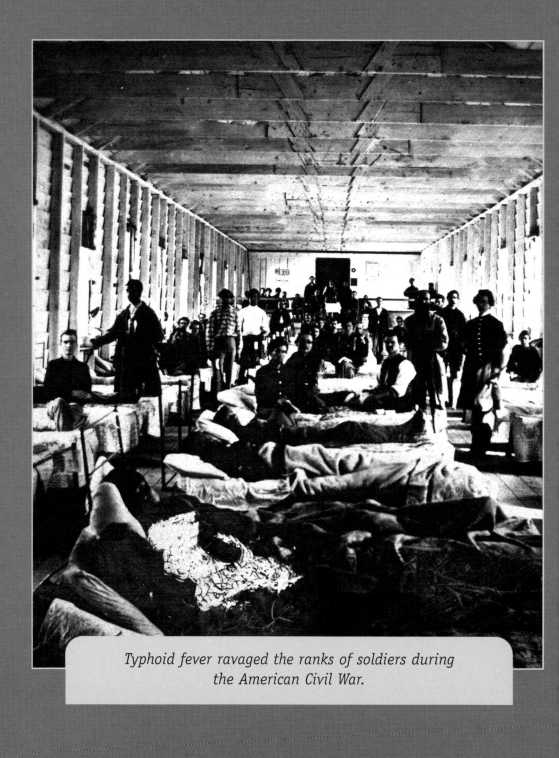

*Typhoid fever ravaged the ranks of soldiers during the American Civil War.*

# INTRODUCTION

Chicago, Illinois, with its growing population, was a quickly developing industrial city in the 1800s. The people who lived in Chicago relied on the waters of nearby Lake Michigan, with its closest source the Chicago River, for drinking, bathing, and farming.

By the 1850s, though, Chicago had a serious water problem that presented residents with a health emergency. Water that was used for drinking was drawn from the same places into which sewage was being dumped. Residents were drinking and washing their hands in water that had also been used to clean the city's toilets. Large industries, such as the Chicago Stockyards, were dumping the bodies of dead animals into the Chicago River. In some

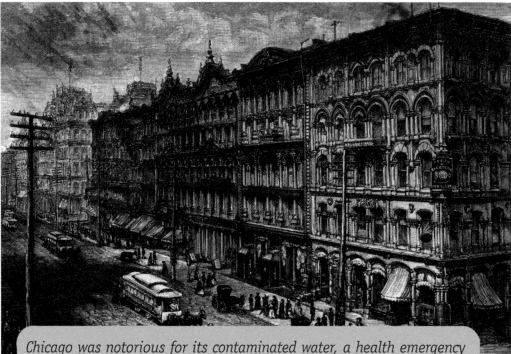

*Chicago was notorious for its contaminated water, a health emergency that forced the city to establish the first commission on sanitation.*

areas, such as a section of the waterway known as Bubbly Creek, the river was so contaminated that the water fermented, giving off the odors of rotting animal flesh.

People who lived in Chicago became very sick. Many residents who drank the water fell ill with terrible headaches and fevers. They lost their appetites and sometimes suffered from severe diarrhea. Some of these people recovered, but they then experienced the same symptoms over again. Many others died. The cause of this sickness and death was typhoid fever.

The fact that people were becoming sick from contaminated water, however, did not stop the city from growing. Chicago was well on its way to becoming the largest port in the United States. By 1881, the disease reached epidemic proportions when 568 people died from typhoid. Throughout the 1880s, thousands of Chicago's residents succumbed to typhoid fever, more than any other area of the United States. Chicago became known as "Typhoid Fever City."

Typhoid fever was, and still is, a problem for people all over the world. We now know what causes typhoid, and we have methods of successfully treating its symptoms. This book tells the story of typhoid fever: what it is, how it is treated, and how we can prevent new infections from occurring.

# 1

# WHAT IS TYPHOID FEVER?

In order to understand a disease such as typhoid fever, you must first understand that diseases originate from bacteria, which are single-celled microorganisms. (The word "micro" means very small, and organisms are living creatures.) In essence, bacteria are incredibly tiny creatures that can be seen only with a microscope.

There are many kinds of bacteria, and each is unique. If you examined many different types of bacteria under a microscope, they would each look very different. Some bacteria are round, others are straight, and still others have shapes that curve. Your own body is composed of millions of different cells, such as skin cells, hair cells, muscle cells, and so on. Unlike your body, bacteria have only one cell.

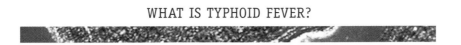

Bacteria are all around us. Some bacteria live in soil or in water. Others live on plants. Bacteria can exist on almost any surface you can think of—a lake, a cutting board, a plant leaf, or your skin.

Bacteria usually live in groups and multiply by cell division, during which the single-celled microorganism splits into two exact parts. Then each of the newly created bacteria divides into two again, and so on. The bacteria continue dividing and multiplying.

Some bacteria are useful and can help plants in the production of oxygen during photosynthesis, the process by which green plants use light to synthesize carbon dioxide. Other bacteria help dead animals decompose once they have died. Because they can multiply so quickly, it can be hard to stop bacteria from increasing and spreading.

## Typhoid Bacteria

Bacteria are divided into groups. Some of the commonly known bacterial groups are *Streptococcus* and *Salmonella*. You probably have heard of streptococcus—the type of bacteria that can cause a terribly sore throat. *Salmonella typhi* is the name of the kind of bacteria (or strain) that causes typhoid fever. There are more than 100 different kinds of *Salmonella typhi* around the world.

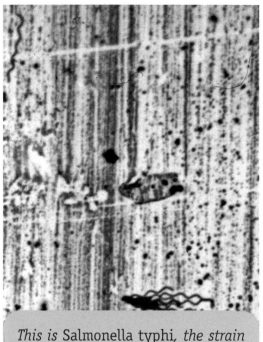

This is Salmonella typhi, the strain of bacteria that causes typhoid fever.

The bacterium *Salmonella typhi* lives inside humans. When someone is infected, the bacterium lives and multiplies in his or her bloodstream and digestive tract (home to the stomach and intestines). The bacteria can be spread to others when an infected person passes feces (also known as stool) out of his or her body. If that feces comes into contact with water that is later used for other purposes, such as cooking or drinking, then anyone who uses that water can become infected with the *Salmonella typhi* bacteria.

This is why people are urged to wash their hands with soap and hot water after using the rest room and before handling food items. Washing with soap kills the bacteria *Salmonella typhi* and helps keep it from spreading.

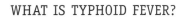

# Sewage Safety

In most of the United States and Europe, we have advanced sewage systems. Sewage is waste material from toilets and sinks, or waste material from businesses. Sewage is treated or dumped, but it is carried in separate pipes from those that bring us clean water for drinking and bathing. Keeping the waste material separate from our drinking water keeps us safe from infection by *Salmonella typhi*.

In many other countries, sewage is handled differently. Many countries are too poor to have advanced sewage systems that keep their wastewater separate from their drinking water. In Africa and Asia, for instance, many larger cities have sewage systems in place, but smaller towns and villages may have only one source of water, such as a nearby lake or river. Some people have no choice but to get their water for drinking and cooking from the same place that they wash their clothes or go to the bathroom. Drinking that contaminated water puts them at risk for infection with *Salmonella typhi*.

Contaminated water can have other adverse effects, too. Fish that live in the tainted water can carry the bacteria on their scales and in their flesh, and later that bacteria may be eaten by humans. Any kind of seafood that comes from water polluted with

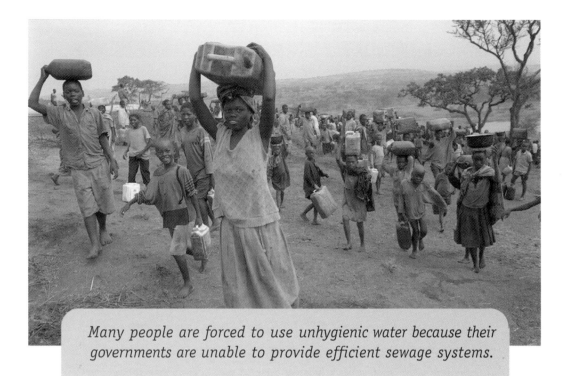

*Many people are forced to use unhygienic water because their governments are unable to provide efficient sewage systems.*

*Salmonella typhi* may be infectious. Even vegetables can be infected, since they sometimes grow in areas near human waste or in contaminated water.

## The Symptoms and Effects of Typhoid Fever

Once someone drinks water or eats food that is contaminated by *Salmonella typhi*, the bacterium develops inside his or her body and begins to multiply. Bacteria enter the bloodstream and travel through the digestive system, including the intestines, the liver, the spleen, and the gallbladder.

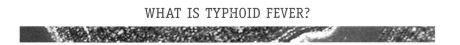

It may take from one to three weeks for someone to begin showing symptoms of typhoid fever after he or she has been infected. In some cases, it can take as long as three months.

The symptoms of typhoid fever are usually most severe after the initial infection. At first, the infected person may think he or she has contracted the flu or a severe cold. An intense headache is followed by a fever and body aches. The fever can get very high (about 104° F), but the person's heart rate is often slowed, which is quite different from a common fever. Nausea (feeling sick to your stomach) and vomiting can occur. Diarrhea is also common. In some cases, infected people get rosy spots on their chests, backs, or stomachs. Inside the body, the spleen and the liver become enlarged.

People who are infected with typhoid fever pass some of the bacteria out of their bodies in their feces each time they have a bowel movement. This process is known as shedding the bacteria. In some cases, infected people shed bacteria in both their urine and their feces. Each time they shed bacteria, there is a possibility that other people can become infected.

In very mild cases, it may be possible for an infected person to shed the bacteria from his or her system completely, without the need for medical treatment. Usually, however, that person's recovery is only temporary. *Salmonella typhi* stays in his or her body and continues to multiply. This can cause recurring health problems. An infected person who survives without treatment will continue to have symptoms from time to time. If typhoid fever is left untreated for long periods, complications such as kidney failure, intestinal bleeding, or peritonitis can result. Eventually, his or her digestive organs will not be able to function correctly, and he or she may die.

## Carriers

A small number of people who are infected by typhoid bacteria may become long-term carriers of the disease. These people recover well enough to continue with day-to-day living, or their symptoms may have been so mild that they did not even realize they were sick. Nonetheless, carriers continue to shed *Salmonella typhi* in their feces and present a constant danger to others with whom they come into contact. If no preventive measures are taken, these people may continue to infect others. Very often these individuals are unaware that they are carriers, which may put those around them at even greater risk.

Although the popular belief is that the ancient leader Alexander the Great (356–324 BC) died of malaria, a disease caused by the bite of infected mosquitos, research now suggests that he actually died of typhoid fever. Research published in the *New England Journal of Medicine* in 1998 reported the symptoms of the dying thirty-two-year-old ruler. They included chills, sweats, exhaustion, and a high fever. History also states that he suffered from severe abdominal pain, a typical symptom of a typhoid infection. The new theory about Alexander's death came about when symptoms that were recorded by ancient historians were analyzed by doctors.

## From Infection to Epidemic

By the 1880s, Chicago's residents had resorted to "water wagons" to haul clean water from nearby Lake Michigan, but the incidence of typhoid cases still reached epidemic proportions. Even though new antidumping laws had been established, the Chicago River was already fully contaminated with raw sewage and the carcasses of dead animals. Many people were still getting their drinking water from the same areas where wastewater was being dumped. As a result, the water supply was contaminated, and thousands of the city's residents were exposed.

Chicago's story illustrates how one person's infection can spread to hundreds or even thousands of people, causing many to be infected with the same disease at around the same time in a place where it is not normally prevalent. This situation is known as an epidemic.

Typhoid fever is not the only disease that has been spread through epidemics. Throughout history, there have been epidemics of deadly diseases such as plague, cholera, and AIDS. Sometimes a population is attacked by more than one epidemic at the same time. During the typhoid fever epidemic in Chicago, for instance, the city was also facing epidemics of smallpox and dysentery. What makes epidemics so dangerous is that they are quick to spread and very difficult to control.

It was during the late nineteenth century that scientists began studying epidemics. The job of these scientists was—and still is—to act as "disease detectives," by searching for clues to the source of an infection. By identifying the infection's source, they try to protect people from it. These scientists are known as epidemiologists.

# The Importance of Hygiene

As a child, you were probably told to wash your hands after going to the bathroom and before every meal. This practice of clean living is called hygiene, which means "healthful." Washing your hands is an important part of good hygiene. As you read about typhoid fever, you can understand why it is so important to keep bacteria from coming into contact with food or drinking water.

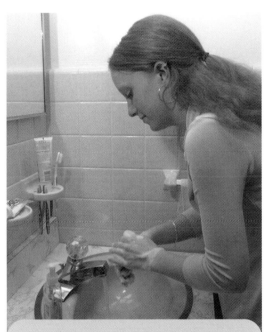

*You should wash frequently with soap and water to kill any dangerous bacteria.*

Remember, it is not just water that can carry the typhoid bacteria. *Salmonella typhi* can be carried on someone's hands and can then be transferred to food or dishes. When you wash your hands with soap and water, the soap often contains ingredients that kill bacteria. Good hygiene is the best method of preventing typhoid fever and many other bacterial diseases.

# 2

# CENTURIES OF DISEASE

Long before Europeans began their explorations of North and South America, typhoid fever was infecting thousands of people in European cities such as Paris and Vienna. No sewage systems existed on a large scale until the nineteenth century, so cities built before that time were stench-ridden, dirty places. In these areas, the lack of clean living conditions allowed *Salmonella typhi* to thrive. In rich and poor areas, living conditions were less than sanitary. Wealthy people had private sitting toilets that emptied into streams or holes in the ground while others used bedpans called chamber pots that were emptied outdoors by servants. Other people had to make do by squatting down next to a tree, on the street, or in a river. With so much human waste in the water and in the soil, the risk of typhoid infection was increased.

# A Deadly Weapon

The known history of typhoid fever dates back to the sixteenth century. During the 1500s, Spanish explorers and soldiers took control of large portions of Mexico and South America in their quest for gold and silver. Spanish leaders such as Francisco Pizarro and Hernán Cortés led their men into bloody battles against Native Americans. Spanish cannons, horses, and guns were much more powerful than Native American spears. However, although the Spanish were not aware of it, they brought with them an even more dangerous weapon: disease.

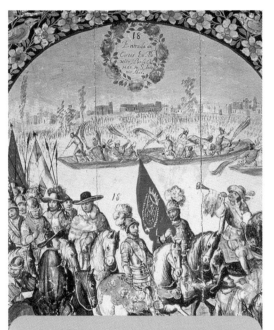

*Spanish conquistadors exposed Native Americans to many bacteria, including typhoid fever.*

Before the Spanish arrived, Native Americans had never been exposed to many of the diseases that were killing Europeans. Typhoid fever was only one of these deadly infections. Cholera, plague, and sexually transmitted infections such as syphilis were also new threats to their lives. Tens of thousands of Native

**Pre-1500**
Typhoid fever is one of many mysterious illnesses in Europe.

**1500s**
Spanish explorers bring typhoid fever and other infectious diseases to the Americas.

**1798**
Edward Jenner creates the first vaccine.

**1860s**
Thousands of Civil War troops die from typhoid fever.

**1607**
The settlers in Jamestown, Virginia, are plagued by typhoid fever, malaria, and starvation.

**1851**
William Jenner identifies typhoid as a separate disease from typhus.

Americans became ill and died as a result of their exposure to European diseases such as typhoid fever. In 1576, an outbreak of typhoid fever in Mexico killed nearly two million people!

# Early American Epidemic

Typhoid fever was brought to North America by European settlers in the 1600s, and perhaps even earlier. English settlers founded the original Jamestown, Virginia, settlement near the banks of the James River on May 13, 1607. Jamestown, which was surrounded on three sides by water, was thought to be an isolated spot

**1880**
Karl Erberth identifies *Salmonella typhi* as the cause of typhoid fever.

**1898**
The U.S. surgeon general orders the creation of the Typhoid Commission.

**1998**
Cases of typhoid fever in Miami, Florida, are attributed to fruit.

**1897**
Almroth Wright creates the first typhoid fever vaccine.

**1907**
"Typhoid Mary" Mallon is quarantined after twenty-two typhoid infections are linked to her.

**1928**
Alexander Fleming accidentally discovers penicillin.

and also one that was easily defendable. The men built a fort and began farming tobacco, drawing the necessary drinking water and irrigation from the James River, the same place where they deposited their wastewater. They firmly believed that the strong river current would wash away the feces and other waste materials, as was the case in London's Thames River.

Unfortunately, the early settlers were wrong. As infected settlers shed *Salmonella typhi* in their feces, it contaminated the river. In summer, the water current slowed, so there was even less chance of the waste being washed away. The bacteria reinfected the settlers each time they drank the infected water.

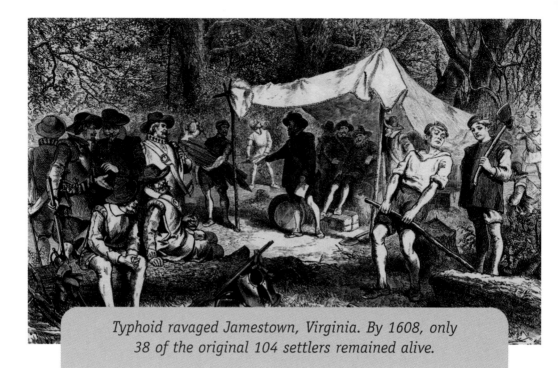

*Typhoid ravaged Jamestown, Virginia. By 1608, only 38 of the original 104 settlers remained alive.*

George Percie, an original Jamestown settler, remarked, "Our drink—cold water taken out of the river, which was at a flooded [state], very salty, and at low tide, full of slime and filth—was the [source of] destruction for many of our men."

As a result, deaths from typhoid fever and other infectious diseases nearly leveled the population of Jamestown on more than one occasion. By the fall season of the first year, nearly one-third of the settlers had already died of disease or of malnutrition. Scholars now speculate that typhoid fever thrived in the swampy Jamestown settlement and was responsible for more than 6,000 deaths of European settlers between 1607 and 1624.

# The Age of Industrialization

During the 1700s and 1800s, industrial growth in American cities began causing problems with waste and disease that European cities had experienced for centuries. As had been done for years, waste was disposed of in the same places from which people drew their drinking water. Raw sewage was thrown out onto the streets and left to rot. Descriptions of Washington, D.C., in the 1860s recall streets and alleys laden with piles of garbage, pigs and other live-stock roaming freely, and vermin inhabiting most dwellings, including the White House. The fumes of rotting sewage were nauseating in a time when people still held fast to the belief that typhoid fever was the result of breathing in the foul gases (then known as miasma) that rose from garbage and sewers. Not surprisingly, typhoid fever was a major cause of death in the United States during this period.

Things worsened during the American Civil War. Cities that were already filthy became even dirtier as large numbers of men headed off to battle. There simply weren't enough people to do the work of keeping things clean or getting rid of garbage. The Potomac River in Washington, D.C., was so polluted by garbage and feces that President Lincoln became ill after eating its fish.

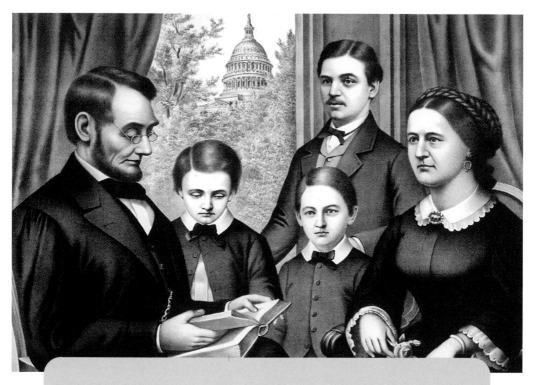

*President Abraham Lincoln's son was the only child ever to die in the White House when he succumbed to typhoid fever in 1862.*

Typhoid fever also affected President Lincoln's family. By 1861, the president, his wife, and their sons, Willie and Tad, moved into the White House. Willie was a smart young man, very likable, an excellent student, and deeply loved by his family. Just after his eleventh birthday on December 21, Willie became very ill with typhoid fever. He became more and more sick until he finally died on February 20, 1862. President Lincoln and his wife were devastated.

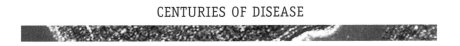

# The Civil War

The Lincolns' experience was not very different from that of many American families at the time. As young men joined the Union and Confederate armies, they were actually in more danger of dying from typhoid fever and other diseases then they were of being killed in battle.

The soldiers' camps often had an area for the men to go to the bathroom, but it was usually on the banks of a river where those same men went to drink. Rainstorms caused these areas to flood, and feces would often overflow and run back into the soldiers' camps. Of all the dangers faced by the soldiers of the Union and Confederate armies, contaminated water posed the worst threat. In a description about the state of the army's drinking water, a Texas surgeon remarked, "We had an awful time drinking the meanest water not fit for a horse (indeed, I could hardly get my horse to drink it)."

Thousands of men became ill with typhoid fever during the Civil War. In fact, it is now estimated that diseases such as typhoid, malaria, pneumonia, and dysentery took the lives of more than 200,000 men while the war raged on until 1865. Surgeons, most working under very extreme circumstances, sometimes

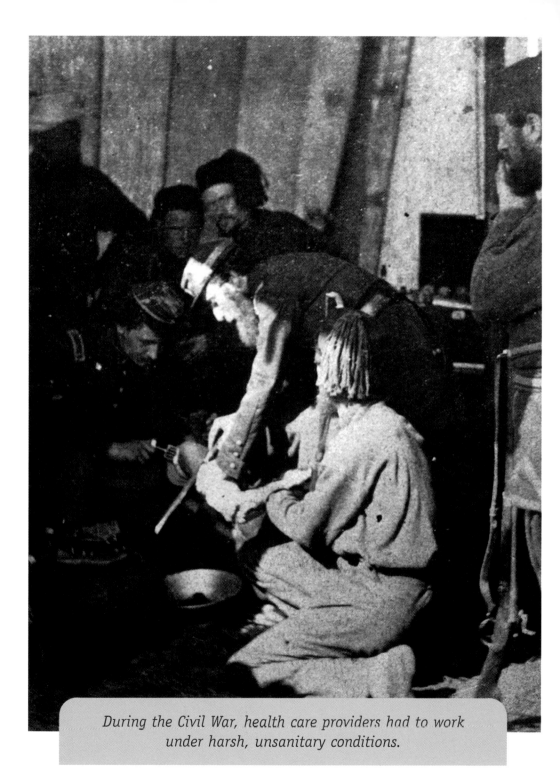

*During the Civil War, health care providers had to work under harsh, unsanitary conditions.*

went for days without the opportunity to wash their hands with clean water and soap; in other foul conditions, vermin such as lice, mites, and fleas spread disease easily from soldier to soldier. Even men who recovered well enough to fight again were still shedding *Salmonella typhi* in their feces, so the cycle of contamination continued.

Following the war, the surgeon general of the United States ordered the first Typhoid Commission to study the causes of typhoid fever and to recommend a disease prevention program for the army.

# Scientific Breakthroughs

Fortunately for the members of the Typhoid Commission, scientific progress was allowing them to track typhoid fever more easily. In 1851, English scientist William Jenner was able to separate the symptoms of typhoid fever from those of typhus. (Typhus was a disease carried by lice that was often confused with typhoid.) In 1880, German scientist Karl Erberth identified *Salmonella typhi* as the cause of typhoid fever. Scientists now knew exactly which bacteria they were searching for.

However, there were many problems ahead. Scientists were only beginning to realize that poor hygiene was the cause of many diseases.

In 1896, while battling a typhoid infection, Orville Wright asked his brother Wilbur to read to him about the death of a famous German glider pilot. After the brothers invented the first airplane, Orville credited this story as initially sparking his interest in flying. Much later, quite ironically (and tragically), his brother Wilbur died of typhoid fever.

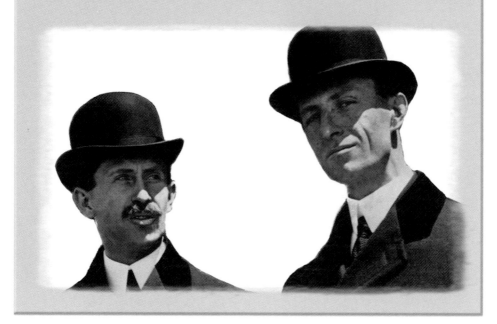

## The Typhoid Commission

The members of the Typhoid Commission were high-ranking surgeons from the U.S. Army. They began their work in 1898, when the death rate from typhoid was more than 800 per every 100,000 soldiers. The commission's job was to recommend ways that U.S. soldiers could be protected from all diseases. Their first challenge was to arrange for every army hospital to have access to equipment, such as microscopes, that would allow them to better study disease.

The Typhoid Commission visited army camps that had suffered from typhoid epidemics. In Chickamauga Park, Georgia, the commission examined a large area where more than 60,000 soldiers had camped during training exercises. What the commission saw shocked them. The ground at Chickamauga Park was very rocky, so the soldiers had not been able to dig holes to use as toilets. Instead, the soldiers left piles of feces on the ground, often several inches high. The park had gotten so crowded that some soldiers were forced to set up their tents in the same area where the waste was piled. A stream that soldiers used for drinking water was also being used as a toilet.

The commission also noticed that men who ate their meals in screened tents developed fewer cases of typhoid fever. The human waste littering the crowded camp attracted thousands of flies. As an experiment, they covered the waste with powdered limestone and watched as the flies landed on the white powder. They then visited the camp's kitchen tents. As flies landed on the food in the kitchen, they left tiny white footprints directly on the food items. In this way, the commission was able to demonstrate that flies were contributing to the spread of typhoid bacteria. Flies and other insects were transporting typhoid bacteria directly from the human waste piles to the food supply. After examining some flies under a microscope, the scientists were able to prove that they carried *Salmonella typhi*.

# Daily Hygiene

The commission continued to study the daily behavior of the soldiers at Chickamauga Park. Each day, some of the men were chosen to work as orderlies in the camp hospital. The orderlies spent time cleaning out bedpans of patients who were sick with typhoid fever. Sometimes the orderlies were careless and slopped human waste wherever they walked. At mealtimes, many of the orderlies went straight to the mess hall to eat without washing.

The commission also noticed that the place where men used the bathroom was too close to the sleeping tents. Most soldiers in Chickamauga Park had to walk through the piles of waste in order to get to another part of the camp. The feces came into contact with their boots and, finally, with tents, beds, and clothing.

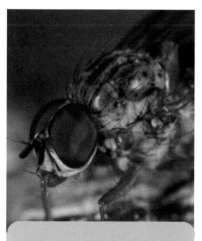

*Flies carry many diseases.*

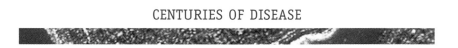

The commission made the decision to treat typhoid fever as a contagious disease. This meant that everything that came into contact with human waste had to be cleaned and disinfected. Everything was washed, including tents, boots, and bedding. Almost immediately, fewer typhoid infections appeared in the camp.

## A Change for the Better

The work of the Typhoid Commission changed the way the army dealt with typhoid fever. Army camps became much cleaner, and as a result, the number of typhoid infections continued to decrease. By 1907, less than ten years after the commission had started its work, the death rate from typhoid infection reached an all-time low: only nineteen deaths per 100,000 soldiers. The Typhoid Commission had succeeded in making the army a safer place to live and work.

# 3

# THE STORY OF TYPHOID MARY

Though the Typhoid Commission made great progress, there was still much work to be done. The general public had not yet learned about the benefits of hygiene. As the twentieth century began, many American cities had sewage systems in place. They were also using basic water filtration systems that eliminated some harmful bacteria, including *Salmonella typhi*. Many private homes had sitting toilets and basic plumbing.

Outbreaks of typhoid fever still occurred frequently. More than 35,000 Americans died from typhoid fever in 1900, keeping citizens at great risk.

## Mary Mallon

In the late 1800s, a young woman named Mary Mallon moved to New York City from Ireland. Like many immigrant women, Mary went to work for wealthy families as a servant. She found success as a cook, and many families recommended her services.

In the summer of 1906, Mary went to work for the Warren family in Oyster Bay, Long Island. The Warrens were renting a house for the season. In total there were eleven people in the Warren household, both family members and servants. During Mary's employment, six of the eleven people—three family members and three servants—became ill with typhoid fever. Since Mary remained healthy, she went to work for another family in upstate New York after the season ended.

## George Soper

Following the outbreak of typhoid in the Warren household, the owners of the house wanted to find out what had caused the epidemic. They asked George Soper, a sanitation engineer, to help them identify the problem. Soper had experience as an epidemiologist, a doctor who studies the spread of disease. He began by checking possible sources of typhoid infection, such as the water and food supply. These sources seemed free of typhoid bacteria, so he began investigating each member of the household.

While interviewing the Warren family, Soper learned that Mary Mallon had come to work for them shortly before the outbreak. About ten days after her arrival, the first person had become sick with typhoid. Almost immediately, Soper felt that Mary's arrival was important. He suspected that Mary was the source of the typhoid infection and was spreading it to others through her cooking.

## Tracing Mary's Steps

George Soper thought that Mary Mallon could be the cause of the typhoid infection in the Warren house, but first he had to prove it. To do this, Soper sought the assistance of Mary's employment agency. Using employment records, Soper began to track down other families for whom Mary had worked. He interviewed other family members, just as he had spoken to the Warrens. What Soper learned from his meetings was amazing.

Between 1900 and 1904, before the period of time when she cooked for the Warrens, Mary Mallon had worked for four other families. In each household where she worked, people became sick with typhoid fever. The cases of typhoid were not unusual by

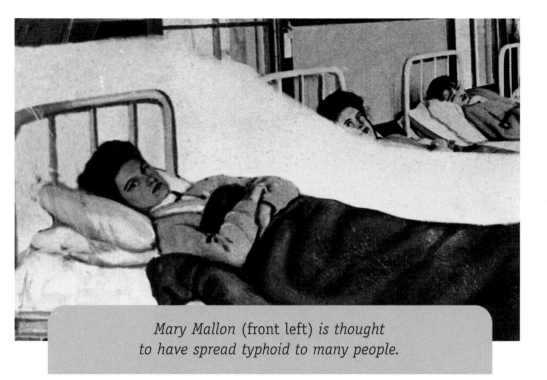

*Mary Mallon* (front left) *is thought to have spread typhoid to many people.*

themselves since the disease was still very common in New York City, but each of the outbreaks of typhoid in these families occurred after Mary Mallon had arrived. Sometimes the typhoid outbreak happened within a month of her arrival. In other cases, it took nearly a year.

There was no evidence of Mary herself ever being ill with typhoid fever, however. Her employment record was excellent, and many of the families praised her for her efforts. Still, Soper felt certain that Mary was the cause of the infections. As an epidemiologist, he knew that it was possible for people to be carriers of disease, even if they showed no symptoms of the infection.

Soper then investigated Mary's employment after she left the Warren household. At her next place of employment, one of the servants became sick, but it was not clear if his illness was typhoid fever. In the winter of 1906, Mary went to work for a wealthy family in New York City. Shortly after her arrival, two members of the Park Avenue household became ill. Then one of them died. Soper knew he needed to act quickly.

## To Catch a Carrier

George Soper had now traced twenty-two cases of typhoid fever to Mary Mallon. In order to prove that she was also infected with typhoid, Soper needed samples of her blood, feces, and urine. These samples would have to be examined under a microscope to see if they contained *Salmonella typhi*. Soper decided to ask Mary for her cooperation with his research.

By March of the following year, 1907, George Soper entered the home where Mary was employed as a cook. He met with her briefly and told her that she was carrying a deadly disease. He asked her for samples of her feces and urine. Mary was upset and confused. She ordered Soper out of the house.

Soper had no power to force Mary to give the samples, so he went to the New York City Health Department. Based on Soper's detective work, the board of health agreed that Mary Mallon was probably the cause of the typhoid infections. They sent a health inspector to help Soper get the samples he needed to prove Mary was carrying *Salmonella typhi* in her system.

Again, Mary refused to cooperate. The health inspector requested help from the police, and Mary was forced to go to a hospital for patients with contagious diseases. At the hospital, she gave samples of her blood, feces, and urine. After the examination of the samples, Soper's theory was proved correct. Every sample contained high levels of *Salmonella typhi*.

## Against Her Will

The city of New York felt it had to keep Mary Mallon away from the rest of its population. The levels of *Salmonella typhi* in her body were so high that she was considered a danger to healthy people. As a result, Mary was forced to live in a cottage near Riverside Hospital in the Bronx. Both the cottage and Riverside Hospital, which specialized in the treatment of infectious diseases, were located on North

Brother Island in the East River. Mary remained quarantined on the island for the next two years. Because of the unusual nature of containment, newspapers tagged her with the nickname "Typhoid Mary."

During her time in the cottage, Mary was instructed to provide samples of her feces every week. The city measured her body's levels of *Salmonella typhi* and used the test results to confine her to the island. Aggravated that her civil rights were being violated, Mary hired a lawyer and sued the city. She wanted to be released. Finally, in 1910, she agreed to never again work as a cook. Upon this agreement, New York City released her from North Brother Island.

At first, Mary kept her end of the agreement and found work as a laundress. Eventually, though, Mary returned to her original occupation as a cook, this time using a false name.

In 1915, the Sloane Maternity Hospital suffered an outbreak of twenty-five cases of typhoid fever. The infection was traced to their cook, Mrs. Brown. "Mrs. Brown" was really Mary Mallon.

Sadly, the city of New York took Mary back to the cottage on North Brother Island. For the next eighteen years, she worked in the laboratories at Riverside Hospital. North Brother Island was Mary's home until her death in 1938 at the age of sixty-nine.

# 4

# IN SEARCH OF A CURE

Typhoid fever had infected humans for centuries before any progress was made toward finding a cure. As science learned about bacteria and other microorganisms, it became easier to find ways to control typhoid fever. Even with the many drugs available today, typhoid remains a deadly disease in many parts of the world, especially in developing countries.

## Learning What Typhoid Is Not

In 1851, William Jenner, an English scientist, identified the symptoms of typhoid fever as separate from those of other deadly diseases. Jenner's work was significant because it proved that typhoid fever was different from typhus, a disease that is carried by insects such as lice and fleas. Both diseases were very common in Europe, and the early symptoms of both diseases—headache and fever—were similar. As typhus progresses, however, it affects the body very differently than typhoid fever. Typhus attacks the heart, lungs, and even the brain, while typhoid fever remains concentrated in the gastrointestinal system.

Thirty years later, a major breakthrough was made. In 1880, a German scientist named Karl Erberth examined *Salmonella typhi* under a microscope. In doing so, Erberth identified exactly which bacteria caused typhoid fever. Other scientists around the world used Erberth's findings to help them begin fighting the typhoid bacteria, too. Erberth's other contribution was to continue what Jenner had begun. Erberth was able to link the specific symptoms of typhoid fever to the *Salmonella typhi* bacteria that caused them in the human body.

# Paratyphoid Fever

There are at least 107 different strains of the *Salmonella typhi* bacteria in the world today. All of these strains infect the body with typhoid fever. Other bacteria in the Salmonella family, such as *Salmonella paratyphoid*, cause milder symptoms that are usually much less dangerous. Infection with *Salmonella paratyphoid* is known as paratyphoid fever, a disease that usually responds to the same treatment as typhoid fever, but one in which deaths are rare. While the process of shedding the bacteria is the same for both infections, the body recovers more easily from paratyphoid fever.

## No Treatment for Typhoid

There was no specific treatment for typhoid fever for thousands of years. Doctors could only try to make a patient comfortable or suggest methods to reduce a person's fever, such as drinking fluids and resting. As the fever rose and the person's other symptoms worsened, there was no treatment available. If he or she was lucky, enough bacteria would be shed from his or her body to reduce the severity of the disease. Sometimes the patient would feel well enough to go back to his or her daily life and activities. Frequently, though, the symptoms would return. In many cases, the patient did not recover: He or she died after a long and very painful illness.

Even more frightening than the symptoms of typhoid fever was the fact that it was extremely contagious. Whenever someone was sick with the disease, everyone in the household was at risk.

For many centuries, humans did not know that bacteria and other organisms caused disease. Many people believed that disease was a curse, or a punishment from God. Because they did not understand what caused disease, they couldn't take steps to prevent it. No one understood that they needed to be careful about the feces of infected people and keeping their food and water supplies clean.

# Vaccines

The twentieth century brought major break-throughs in the treatment and prevention of many diseases that had affected human beings for centuries. One of the most important scientific developments was the widespread use of vaccines. Vaccines are medicines that help the body learn how to fight specific infections.

Vaccines stimulate the immune system, which releases particles in our bodies that fight disease. When an infection from bacteria enters the body, the immune system releases white blood cells known as lymphocytes. The lymphocytes attack the invading infection. When lymphocytes are successful, the body recovers from its symptoms and illness. When they fail, the body continues to suffer from symptoms or is overcome by them and dies.

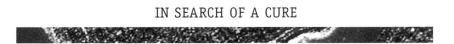

# An Early Vaccine

In 1798, Edward Jenner tried an experiment to fight smallpox. Smallpox was a very contagious disease with a high death rate that was common in England. However, Dr. Jenner noticed that there were some people who did not catch smallpox even when other family members died of the disease. These individuals, he found, had been exposed to another disease called cowpox. (Cowpox was a mild illness that primarily affected people who worked with cattle.)

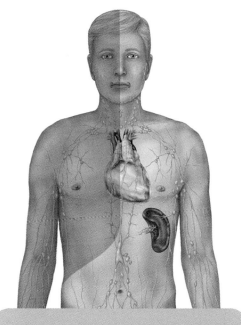

*The immune system contains the lymph nodes, which release particles into the body to fight disease.*

Dr. Jenner hypothesized (made an educated guess) that those who had been infected with cowpox had developed a natural immunity (resistance) to smallpox. To prove his theory, Jenner met with Sarah Nelmes, a milkmaid who had just become infected with cowpox. Sarah had small sores on her fingers from the infection, a common side effect of the disease. Dr. Jenner took some of the matter he squeezed from Sarah's sores and injected it into a seven-year-old boy who had never been infected with either cowpox or smallpox. The boy became slightly ill from the cowpox, but he quickly recovered.

After the boy recovered from cowpox, Dr. Jenner infected him with smallpox. Nothing happened. The boy did not develop any symptoms of a smallpox infection. Dr. Jenner's experiment had proven that infecting people with cowpox protected them from the much more serious infection of smallpox. During the next 100 years, doctors and scientists worked very diligently to find vaccines for other diseases in this same manner. They also tried other methods of vaccination, such as infecting people with weakened bacteria from the very disease they were fighting.

## The Typhoid Vaccine

In 1897, British scientist Almroth Wright developed a vaccine against typhoid fever. Wright took *Salmonella typhi* bacteria and allowed it to multiply in a controlled laboratory setting. Next, he took the bacteria and preserved it in a solution. Finally, he heated the solution to a high temperature that killed the bacteria. The *Salmonella typhi* in the solution died. What was left was a solution that contained dead typhoid bacteria.

When the solution was injected into humans, the body reacted as if the bacteria were alive. The body then released lymphocytes to fight the infection. Sometimes the person who was vaccinated developed mild symptoms, but they were not nearly as serious as the effects of typhoid infection from contaminated water or food. More important, vaccination allowed the body to develop immunity to the disease. If faced with infection from live *Salmonella typhi*, the body could fight the disease on its own.

Wright's typhoid vaccine was a big breakthrough. The vaccine was used to protect British soldiers who were stationed in India, a country with a very high

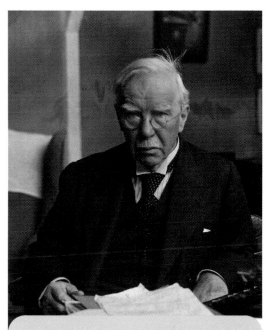

*Almroth Wright developed a vaccine against typhoid fever.*

rate of typhoid infection. During World War I, the British troops were the only soldiers who were vaccinated against typhoid fever. By 1911, it became a standard procedure to vaccinate American soldiers, too.

# Antibiotics

The next breakthrough in the treatment of typhoid fever was the discovery of antibiotics. Antibiotics (from the word "anti," meaning against, and "biotics," meaning living organisms) are medicines that kill bacteria. They are usually made from chemicals that are released by other microorganisms.

Alexander Fleming discovered the first antibiotic in 1928. Fleming was a Scottish scientist who accidentally left a dish of bacteria out on his laboratory table. Several days later, he saw that a mold, later called *Penicillium notatum*, had grown across the top of the dish. When he examined it under a microscope, Fleming realized that the mold had killed the bacteria. He named the new antibiotic penicillin.

Based on Fleming's discovery, other scientists focused their work on finding antibiotics like penicillin. Even today, when new bacterial infections are identified, scientists search for antibiotics to fight them. There are several antibiotics that are currently used to fight typhoid fever. Two of the most common are amoxicillin and chloramphenicol. Both of these antibiotic drugs should be used only when prescribed by a doctor. If not used carefully, they may have dangerous side effects that can affect bone marrow or even kill younger patients.

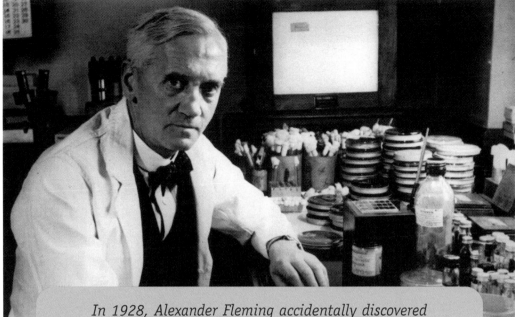

*In 1928, Alexander Fleming accidentally discovered the first antibiotic, penicillin.*

# Drug Resistance

Even though modern science has developed antibiotics and vaccines to fight disease, bacteria such as *Salmonella typhi* are always changing. There are currently more than 100 strains of typhoid bacteria, and they do not all respond to the same antibiotics. Vaccinations that protect against some of the strains may not protect against all of them.

Another problem is drug resistance. Drug resistance occurs when a bacteria begins to adapt to the medicine that is being used to kill it. Chloramphenicol is one of the antibiotics that is used to fight *Salmonella typhi*.

Unfortunately, even the best antibiotic doesn't kill all the bacteria. Remaining bacteria survive with a resistance to chloramphenicol. After the resistant bacteria multiply during the normal process of cell division, there are more and more bacteria with the same resistance to that drug. If the resistant bacteria infect a new person, then that infection is resistant to chloramphenicol. In cases such as this, a different drug will have to be used to fight the disease.

Drug resistance is not only a problem when fighting typhoid fever. Drug resistance occurs in hundreds of different diseases, including malaria, AIDS, and pneumonia, to name only a few. Because more people in the world take antibiotics to fight many different kinds of disease, there are more drug-resistant strains of infection developing every year. The danger is that we will run out of medicines that are effective against certain diseases. Though new drugs are being created each year, it would be impossible to keep up with every drug-resistant disease that develops.

## Disease Detectives

For the last 150 years, epidemiologists and public health workers have done important work in fighting typhoid fever. Like George Soper in the case of Mary Mallon, these people act as disease detectives.

When someone is infected with typhoid fever, the epidemiologists try to find the source of the infection. By tracing an infection to its source, they can get treatment for other sick people and prevent new infections from occurring.

Leslie Lumsden was a member of the United States Public Health Service during the early 1900s. He investigated many outbreaks of typhoid fever on the East Coast that came from contaminated milk and water supplies. In 1911, he was sent to Yakima, Washington, where an epidemic of typhoid had lasted nearly three years. Lumsden used his skills to trace the source of infection to unsafe public toilets. In addition to helping the residents of Yakima correct the problem, Lumsden suggested that they start a county health service of their own. As a result, Yakima became the first county in the United States to establish its own public health department.

It is still the job of U.S. public health departments to track outbreaks of disease. The skills that were developed by epidemiologists in the early 1900s are still used today to track not only typhoid, but also herpes, gonorrhea, and other sexually transmitted diseases (STDs). Their job is to help prevent future infections and alert anyone who may have been exposed to a disease without knowing it.

# Water Treatment

By the late 1800s, scientists had proven that *Salmonella typhi* was transmitted through an infected person's feces. They now understood that water supplies had to be kept clean in order to keep the population healthy. This information led to the development of different kinds of water filters. Some of the earliest water filters were made with sand. In a sand filter, water would pass through sand before anyone drank it. The sand held back small particles, like feces and some bacterial organisms, keeping the drinking water much cleaner. Many microorganisms could still pass through the sand, but it was a step in the right direction.

Efforts were then made to use chemicals to kill bacteria in the water. The most successful of these chemicals is still used today: chlorine. Chlorine is added to the water supply in most places that have advanced water filtration systems. In addition to other methods of filtration, chlorine is the final step toward a cleaner, healthier supply of drinking water.

# 5

# A FUTURE WITHOUT TYPHOID?

**W**ith all the advances in science and medicine, is it possible that typhoid fever can be eliminated? It's difficult to realize how great a threat typhoid fever is, since the disease is very rare in the United States. Unfortunately, typhoid fever continues to infect people in great numbers all over the world. In 1995, for instance, there were an estimated 17 million cases of typhoid fever worldwide, with 600,000 deaths resulting from the disease.

## Typhoid Fever Around the World

Though it is rare in the United States, typhoid fever is still a major problem for people in developing countries. In 1999, for instance, an

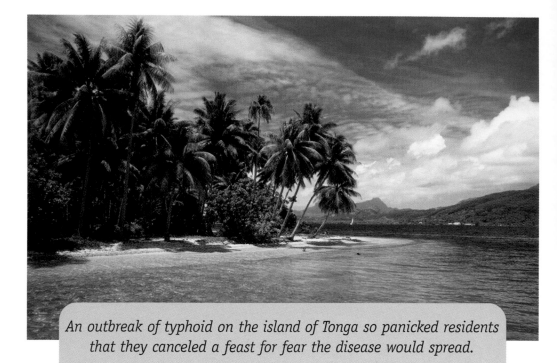

*An outbreak of typhoid on the island of Tonga so panicked residents that they canceled a feast for fear the disease would spread.*

outbreak of typhoid on the Pacific island of Tonga forced the residents to cancel a public feast because of fears that the disease would spread. In Tajikistan, a country that was once a province of the former Soviet Union, typhoid fever is a major health threat. Tajikistan has a very primitive system for sewage and drinking water. As a result, many people become infected with typhoid fever and do not have access to modern medical care. These are just two examples of the hundreds of places facing the threat of infection from *Salmonella typhi* and many other deadly bacteria.

Matthew Curlewis is a successful dancer and performer from Australia. In 1986, at the age of twenty-one, Curlewis traveled alone through China, Tibet, and Nepal. These three countries have very primitive systems for sewage and drinking water, and each has a high rate of typhoid fever infection. After leaving Nepal, Curlewis flew to London to spend time with friends.

After arriving in London, Curlewis noticed that his skin and eyes were yellow. A doctor confirmed that he was suffering from hepatitis (a disease of the liver that can be caught in much the same way as typhoid fever). The doctor felt confident that Curlewis would recover quickly, but his health continued to worsen. Soon he was unable to stay conscious. A worried friend phoned an ambulance, and he was rushed to a London hospital.

For the next several days, Curlewis was in and out of a coma. He began to have seizures. Doctors performed many tests but were unable to identify his illness. When Curlewis began to come out of the coma, he explained to his doctors that he had been traveling in Nepal before coming to London. The doctors then tested Curlewis for *Salmonella typhi*. He tested positive and was moved to a hospital for infectious diseases for seven weeks. Any friends who had shared a meal with Curlewis had to be tested for both typhoid fever and hepatitis. Luckily, they all tested negative.

After seven weeks, there was no evidence of *Salmonella typhi* in his body. Curlewis was allowed to go home. He was still very weak. It took a full year of recovery before he was strong enough to dance again.

There have even been outbreaks much closer to home. In December 1998, the city of Miami began to experience cases of typhoid fever. Florida health workers traced the epidemic to frozen mamey, a fruit that is imported from Central America. After warning consumers not to eat any frozen mamey fruit, the outbreak was eventually traced to a factory in Guatemala that had already been shut down because of safety violations.

# The Future of Hygiene

In 1997, President Bill Clinton proposed spending $43 million to battle food contamination. Even with low rates of typhoid infection in the United States, nearly 9,000 people die each year from different kinds of food poisoning. Many others become sick. In response, one U.S. company has created a machine that sounds an alert if an employee does not wash his or her hands after going to the rest room.

The problems caused by poor personal hygiene affect everyone. While water and food is usually safe, it is still necessary to be aware of possible exposure to typhoid fever. If you may have been exposed to *Salmonella typhi* or another dangerous bacteria, you should see a doctor as quickly as possible. Remember that keeping clean is the best way to battle infection.

- An important guideline for travelers is "Boil it, cook it, peel it, or forget it!"

- If you drink water, bring it to a rolling boil for one minute before you drink it. Bottled carbonated water (with bubbles) is safer than noncarbonated water.

- It is safer to drink a canned or bottled beverage than one from a container that was not known to be clean or dry.

- Water may be consumed if it is treated with iodine or chlorine tablets. These are available at your local sporting goods store or pharmacy.

- Don't ask for drinks with ice unless you know that it has been made from bottled or boiled water.

- Eat foods that have been thoroughly cooked and that are still hot and steaming.

- Avoid eating raw vegetables and fruits that cannot be peeled. Vegetables such as lettuce are easily contaminated and difficult to wash.

- When you eat fruits or vegetables, peel them yourself after washing your hands with soap.

- Avoid food and drink from street vendors. Many travelers have been known to get sick from food bought from street vendors that was not properly prepared.

- Avoid unpasteurized milk products, raw meat, and shellfish.

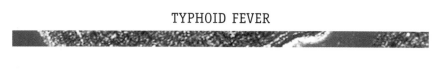

# Protecting Yourself

The best defense against typhoid fever is to avoid coming in contact with it. There are many things that you can do to prevent infection. Since food or water that has been contaminated with feces spreads typhoid fever, it is important to always wash your hands after going to the bathroom. It is equally important to wash your hands before handling food.

The risk of typhoid infection in the United States, Canada, and Europe is extremely low. You are unlikely to come into contact with typhoid fever during your day-to-day life, especially if you live in an area that has modern plumbing and clean, running water. If you are traveling to other parts of the world, however, it is very important to check with your doctor about what steps you can take to protect yourself.

Vacationers are often vaccinated against typhoid fever. When you are vaccinated, your doctor will give you an injection (a shot). Most people experience no side effects from vaccination, but some may have a mild reaction, such as soreness or even a fever. Any side effects should clear up very quickly.

# GLOSSARY

**AIDS**  Disease of the human immune system caused by the human immunodeficiency virus (HIV).

**antibiotics**  Medicines that attack living organisms like bacteria.

**bacteria**  One-celled microorganisms.

**cholera**  Disease of the human digestive system.

**contagious**  Something that can be spread easily.

**contaminated**  Infected or polluted, as in "contaminated water."

**decompose**  To rot.

**dysentery**  Disease that causes severe diarrhea.

**epidemic**  When many people are infected with the same disease at around the same time.

**epidemiology**  Study of epidemics.

**feces**  Human solid waste; also called stool.

**gall bladder**  Organ in the digestive system that stores bile, a substance that aids in digestion.

**hygiene**  Practice of clean living, like washing your hands.

**immune**  Protected from disease.

**infectious**  Something that spreads infection.

**initial**   First.

**paratyphoid fever**   Disease with similar symptoms to typhoid fever; caused by the bacteria *Salmonella paratyphoid*.

**peritonitis**   Infection of the membrane that surrounds the organs of the digestive system.

**photosynthesis**   Process by which green plants convert light, carbon dioxide, and water into oxygen.

**plague**   Disease that causes swelling of the lymph nodes.

*Salmonella typhi*   Bacteria that causes typhoid fever.

**sewage**   Waste matter that is usually carried away by sewer pipes.

**spleen**   Organ in the digestive system that filters red blood cells.

**symptom**   Something that indicates the presence of a disease or another problem within the body.

**typhoid fever**   Disease of the digestive system caused by the bacteria *Salmonella typhi*.

**typhus**   Bacterial disease that is carried by lice.

**vaccine**   Medicine that stimulates the body's immune system.

# FOR MORE INFORMATION

## In the United States

The Centers for Disease Control (CDC)
1600 Clifton Road
Atlanta, GA 30333
(800) 311-3435
(404) 639-3311
Web site: http://www.cdc.gov
The CDC is the federal agency responsible for protecting the health and safety of all people in the United States. The CDC Web site is a great resource for information on infectious diseases of all kinds.

The National Travelers CDC Health Hotline
(877) 394-8747

Lonely Planet
http://www.lonelyplanet.com
Lonely Planet is a publisher of travel guidebooks to all parts of the world.

World Health Organization (WHO)
525 23rd Street NW
Washington, DC 20037
(202) 974-3000
Web site: http://www.who.org

## In Canada

Bureau of Infectious Diseases
Health Protection Branch
Health Canada
Tunney's Pasture
Ottawa, ON K1A 0L2
Web site: http://www.hc-sc.gc.ca

Canadian Medical Association
1867 Alta Vista Drive
Ottawa, ON K1G 3Y6
(888) 855-2555
(800) 663-7336
Web site: http://www.cma.ca

# FOR FURTHER READING

Bourdain, Anthony. *Typhoid Mary: An Urban Historical*. New York: Bloomsbury Publishers, 2001.

Chin, James, ed. *Control of Communicable Diseases Manual*. Washington, DC: American Public Health Association, 2000.

Hoff, Brent, and Carter Smith III. *Mapping Epidemics: A Historical Atlas of Disease*. New York: Franklin Watts, 2000.

Karlen, Arno. *Man and Microbes: Disease and Plagues in History and Modern Times*. New York: Touchstone Books, 1996.

Leavitt, Judith Walzer. *Typhoid Mary: Captive to the Public's Health*. Boston, MA: Beacon Press, 1996.

# INDEX

**A**
AIDS, 16, 48
Alexander the Great, 15
amoxicillin, 46
antibiotics, 46, 47–48

**B**
bacteria, definition/explana-
    tion of, 8–9

**C**
chloramphenicol, 46,
    47–48
chlorine, 50
cholera, 16, 19
Civil War, 23, 25–27
Clinton, President Bill, 54
contaminated water, danger
    of, 11–12, 25, 56
Cortés, Hernán, 19
cowpox, 43–44
Curlewis, Matthew, 53

**D**
drug resistance, 47–48
dysentery, 16, 25

**E**
epidemic, definition of, 16
epidemiologists, 16, 33, 35,
    48, 49
Erberth, Karl, 27, 40

**F**
Fleming, Alexander, 46

**H**
hygiene, importance of, 10,
    17, 27, 54, 56

**I**
immune system, function
    of, 42
industrial growth, problems
    caused by, 23

**J**
Jenner, Edward, 43–44
Jenner, William, 27, 39–40

**L**
Lincoln, President Abraham,
    23–24, 25
Lumsden, Leslie, 49

**M**

malaria, 15, 25, 48
Mallon, Mary (Typhoid
Mary), 33–38, 48
miasma, 23

**N**

Native Americans, 19–20
Nelmes, Sarah, 43–44

**P**

paratyphoid fever, 40–41
penicillin, 46
Percie, George, 22
Pizarro, Francisco, 19
plague, 16, 19
pneumonia, 25, 48

**S**

*Salmonella typhi*
carriers of, 14
explanation of, 9–10,
12–14, 40
scientific identification
of, 27, 40
spread/transfer, 10, 11–12,
13, 17, 27, 30, 50
sexually transmitted
infections, 19, 49
shedding, 13, 14, 21, 27, 41
smallpox, 16, 43–44
Soper, George, 33–37, 48
Spanish explorers, spread of
disease by, 19–20

**T**

Typhoid Commission, 27,
28–31, 32
typhoid fever
carriers of, 14, 35
causes/transmission of,
9–10, 11–12, 13
history of, 18–31
prevention, 17, 42, 55, 56
symptoms, 12–14, 15, 40
treatment for, 41, 46
vaccine for, 44–45, 56
"Typhoid Fever City," 7
typhoid fever outbreaks/
epidemics
Chicago, Illinois, (1880s),
5–7, 15–16
Jamestown, Virginia,
(1607–1624), 20–22
Mexico (1576), 20
Miami, Florida, (1998), 54
Sloane Maternity Hospital,
New York, (1915), 38
Tonga (1999), 52
Yakima, Washington,
(1911), 49
typhus, 27, 39–40

**W**

water treatment/filtration,
32, 50
Wright, Almroth, 44–45
Wright, Orville and Wilbur, 28

# CREDITS

## About the Author

Kurt Ray is a freelance author who has written many books for young adults. He lives in Bozeman, Montana, where he enjoys his passions for fly-fishing and the music of Artaud Filberto.

## Photo Credits

Cover © Tektoff-Merieux, CNRI/Science Photo Library/Photo Researchers, Inc.; p. 4 © Medford Historical Society/Corbis; p. 6 © Corbis; p. 10 © Biophoto Associates/Photo Researchers, Inc.; p. 12 © David and Peter Turnley/Corbis; p. 15 © Araldo de Luca/Corbis; p. 17 by Maura Boruchow; p. 19 © Museo de America/Bridgeman Art Gallery/London Superstock; p. 22, 28, 35 © Bettmann/Corbis; p. 24 © Stock Montage/Archive Photos; p. 26 © Archive Photos; p. 30 © George Lepp/ Corbis; p. 43 © Custom Medical; p. 45 © Hulton-Deutsch/Corbis; p. 47 © Associated Press/AP; p. 52 © Neil Rabinowitz/Corbis.

## Series Design

Evelyn Horovicz

## Layout

Thomas Forget

**DATE DUE**

| OCT 2 0 20 | | | |
|---|---|---|---|
| | | | |
| | | | |
| | | | |
| | | | |
| | | | |
| | | | |
| | | | |
| | | | |
| | | | |
| | | | |
| | | | |
| | | | |
| | | | |
| | | | |
| | | | |
| | | | |
| GAYLORD | | | PRINTED IN U.S.A. |